BALANITIS

A Comprehensive Overview of Inflammation in Males: Balanitis and Beyond

CARL JUAN

Table of Contents

Introductory 4

CHAPTER ONE.....................7

Various Balanitis Forms 7

CHAPTER TWO.....................17

Male Genital Structure and
Performance...............................17

Balanitis and Male
Circumcision 24

CHAPTER THREE.....................28

Leadership That Is
Conservative 28

Alternative Treatments...........33

CHAPTER FOUR.....................39

Balanitis Precautions...............39

Sustaining Balanitis.................44

Conclusion...................................50

THE END.....................53

Introductory

When the rounded tip of the male genitalia, the glans penis, becomes inflamed, a condition known as balanitis, develops. Males who have not had circumcision are more likely to experience this illness, while circumcised men are not immune. There are many potential origins of balanitis, some of which include:

• The collection of smegma, a mixture of dead skin cells and body oils, can irritate the glans and cause inflammation if the vaginal area is not cleaned properly.

• Bacterial or fungal infections are possible causes of balanitis. Inflammation can be caused by a number of factors, including yeast infections like Candida and certain types of bacteria.

• The glans can get inflamed if they come into contact with irritants such as soaps, lotions, or allergies.

• Sexually transmitted diseases (STIs): Herpes and syphilis are two STIs that can cause balanitis.

• When the penile foreskin is too taut, a condition known as phimosis occurs. Because phimosis can trap irritants and bacteria under the foreskin, it can increase the likelihood of balanitis.

Redness, swelling, itching, discomfort, and discharge are all possible symptoms of balanitis. Improved cleanliness, the application of topical antifungal or antibacterial drugs, or, in severe situations, circumcision may be recommended as treatments.

Balanitis and other uncommon genital symptoms warrant a trip to the doctor to rule out more serious conditions and start effective therapy.

CHAPTER ONE
Various Balanitis Forms

Multiple subtypes of balanitis have been identified, each with its own set of symptoms and potential causes. Instances of balanitis include the following:

1. Balanitis of an infectious nature can be brought on by a number of pathogens, such as bacteria, fungi, and viruses. Here are some concrete examples:

• Candidal balanitis is a condition brought on by a yeast infection of the genus Candida, most often Candida albicans.

Results from bacterial infections; Streptococcus and Staphylococcus species are common culprits. o Bacterial balanitis.

• Balanitis brought on by HSV (herpes simplex virus) is called herpetic balanitis. The glans may become sore and ulcerated as a result.

2. Balanitis of the zoon, also known as plasma cell balanitis, is a rare condition characterized by a rash that appears reddish-brown on the glans. The specific reason is unknown, however it is most common in elderly, uncircumcised men.

3. Balanitis of the skin brought on by contact with allergens or irritants is called contact dermatitis. It can be provoked by particular soaps, lotions, latex, or other chemicals.

4. Balanitis caused by trauma to the glans is called traumatic balanitis. Sexual activity can cause inflammation due to friction, abrasions, or injuries.

5. Circinate Balanitis: This is a special kind of balanitis associated with reactive arthritis (Reiter's syndrome). Symptoms include red, achy lesions on the glans and inflammation and pain in the joints.

6. In phimosis, the foreskin is excessively tight and cannot be retracted over the glans, a condition known as phimotic balanitis. Inflammation is caused by microorganisms and sweat that are trapped behind the foreskin when it cannot be pulled back.

7. Balanitis can be divided into two subtypes: erosive and non-erosive. Erosive Balanitis occurs when the glans develop erosions or ulcers as a result of skin problems or autoimmune disorders.

Balanitis treatments are condition specific. Antifungal or antibacterial medication, better cleanliness, treating allergic reactions, and even circumcision are all possible methods. You should see a doctor for a proper diagnosis and treatment of balanitis if you suspect you have it or are experiencing symptoms.

Balanitis symptoms may include, but are not limited to, the following (they may vary according on the underlying cause and the individual):

• There may be redness, swelling, and irritation at the penis's glans (head).

• There may be itching, burning, or general discomfort in the genital area.

• **Pain or Soreness:** Pain in the glans or foreskin may occur, especially during urination or sexual activity.

• Some forms of balanitis are associated with a discharge that might be white, yellow, or green in color.

• Balanitis can cause rashes, blisters, ulcers, or lesions on the glans, depending on the underlying reason.

• Those with balanitis who have bacterial or fungal infections may detect a putrid odor.

• Phimotic balanitis has been linked to difficulty in retracting the foreskin.

• Inflammation can cause pain during urinating if it becomes severe enough.

Balanitis can be diagnosed by a comprehensive examination by a doctor, usually a urologist or dermatologist, which may involve the following:

1. The patient's medical history, including any prior genital

infections, sexual history, hygiene routines, and exposure to potential irritants, will be thoroughly examined by the healthcare practitioner.

2. Physical Examination: A physical examination of the genital area will be undertaken to assess the level of inflammation, check for discharge, and inspect any obvious signs.

3. If the foreskin is implicated and the patient is not circumcised, the doctor will examine the foreskin to see if it is in good enough shape to be retracted.

4. Tests: Depending on the suspected cause, the doctor may request particular tests, such as a swab or culture to identify the causative organism, blood tests, or other diagnostic procedures to rule out underlying illnesses or sexually transmitted infections.

5. A skin biopsy may be conducted if a definitive diagnosis cannot be made or if an underlying skin problem is suspected.

When the doctor knows what's causing the balanitis, they can provide you advice on how to treat it. Antibiotics can be used to treat bacterial infections, antifungal drugs can treat fungal infections, topical corticosteroids can treat inflammation and irritation, and so on.

Timely diagnosis and treatment can help prevent problems and provide relief from discomfort, so it's crucial to visit a doctor if you suspect you have balanitis or have any of the aforementioned symptoms. Furthermore, some forms of balanitis may be linked to STDs, which may necessitate specialized therapies and partner notification.

CHAPTER TWO
Male Genital Structure and Performance

The male genitalia, commonly known as the male reproductive system, have multiple components with diverse physical features and functions. These organs cooperate to assist urination and reproduction by producing, transporting, and delivering sperm. The male genitalia are described in general terms, including their structure and function, below.

1. A Pair Of Testicles.

• The testes are two oval-shaped organs found in the scrotum, an external skin pouch. The seminiferous tubules in each testis are protected by a fibrous capsule.

The testes' principal role is sperm production (spermatogenesis) and the secretion of testosterone and other male sex hormones.

2. Epididymis:

• The epididymis is a long, coiled tube that attaches to the rear of each testis anatomically.

The epididymis is responsible for sperm storage and development, making them fertile and mobile.

3. The ductus deferens (Vas Deferens):

• The epididymis and the pelvic cavity are connected by a muscle tube called the vas deferens.

• **Function:** It delivers mature sperm from the epididymis to the urethra, where they can be ejaculated during sexual intercourse.

4. Seeds of Potential:

• Anatomically speaking, they are two glands that sit behind the bladder, close to where the bladder's neck begins.

The seminal vesicles produce a viscous, alkaline fluid rich in fructose and prostaglandins, which has a functional purpose. This fluid offers food and energy for sperm and helps reduce the acidity of the uterine lining.

5. Men's Prostate:

• The prostate is a walnut-sized gland that lines the urethra and rests just below the bladder.

The milky, alkaline fluid that makes up most of semen is secreted by the prostate gland. This fluid is vital for the sperm's activation and survival.

6. Cowper's Glands, or the Bulbourethral Glands:

• These glands, about the size of a pea, are found at the bottom of the penis.

• The bulbourethral glands produce a transparent, slippery fluid that lubricates the urethra and neutralizes the acidity left behind by urine, making it more conducive to the successful fertilization of sperm.

7. Urethra:

• The urethra is a conduit that travels from the bladder to the penis and then to the body's exterior.

The urethra is important because it transports both pee and sperm. It removes waste from the urinary bladder and carries sperm from the testes after ejaculation.

8. Penis:

• The penis is the male reproductive organ that protrudes from the body. Two cavernous corpora and a spherical corpus spongiosum make up this structure. The penis's rounded tip, or glans penis, is its defining feature.

- When a man gets sexually aroused, his penis will erect so that it can be put into a woman's vagina. The sperm is released through the urethra of the penis after ejaculation, making its way into the female reproductive system.

Although it also contributes to sexual gratification and urine elimination, the male reproductive system's principal job is in sperm production and delivery for fertilization. Testosterone and other male reproductive hormones play an important role in shaping and sustaining secondary sexual traits and general male well-being.

Balanitis and Male Circumcision

Foreskin (prepuce) removal from the penis (glans) is the surgical operation known as circumcision. Most males undergo circumcision for religious, cultural, or medical reasons. Balanitis is one of several medical diseases for which circumcision is sometimes recommended as a preventative measure.

The link between circumcision and balanitis is best explained by considering the following:

- It has been proven that circumcision can help prevent

balanitis in some people. This is because balanitis can be caused by the collection of smegma (a mixture of dead skin cells and body oils) and the growth of bacteria or fungi, both of which are prevented when the foreskin is removed along with the warm, moist environment beneath it.

• Decreased Possibility of PhimosisForeskin that is too taut to be drawn back over the glans is said to be phobic. Because it can trap irritants and bacteria under the foreskin, this condition can raise the risk of balanitis. Phimosis, which can lead to balanitis, can be avoided with circumcision.

• Although circumcision has been shown to reduce the risk of balanitis, it is important to weigh the dangers with the benefits before deciding whether or not to undergo the surgery. Cultural, religious, and familial considerations can all play a role in a person's decision to undergo circumcision. The potential health benefits and hazards linked with circumcision can be discussed with a doctor.

It's worth noting that even after circumcision, a man can develop balanitis if he has poor hygiene, is exposed to irritants, or is sick. Regardless of whether or not a person has been circumcised, good genital hygiene, particularly regular penis cleaning, is vital in preventing balanitis.

If you or someone you know is having symptoms of balanitis or is considering circumcision, it's advisable to visit a healthcare professional for a comprehensive evaluation, consultation, and appropriate suggestions depending on specific circumstances.

CHAPTER THREE
Leadership That Is Conservative

When referring to medical treatment, the term "conservative management" describes methods that do not involve surgery or other intrusive procedures. Conservative management of balanitis refers to the use of non-invasive treatments for the condition. Some safe methods for dealing with balanitis:

1. Hygiene Practices: Proper genital hygiene is vital in avoiding and managing balanitis. As part of this routine, it's important to routinely cleanse the penis and the area under the foreskin with warm water and mild soap. The collection of smegma, which can irritate the glans and lead to balanitis, can be avoided with careful cleaning and thorough drying.

2. Treatment with topical drugs may be recommended for balanitis, depending on the underlying reason. Here's an example:

Candidal balanitis may require the use of antifungal lotions or ointments.

• **Topical Steroids:** Inflammation and irritation can be treated with topical corticosteroids, which may be given by a doctor for a limited time.

3. Balanitis can be alleviated by avoiding any triggers that could make it worse. Do not use soaps, detergents, or other topical items that are too abrasive on your skin.

4. When a more serious infection is the underlying cause of balanitis, oral drugs such as oral antifungals or antibiotics may be recommended.

5. Balanitis can be avoided if the tight foreskin, or phimosis, is treated with mild stretching exercises and possibly topical steroid creams. A physician may advise circumcision in certain circumstances.

6. It is crucial to identify and avoid allergens or irritants if contact dermatitis is suspected. This may require modifying the type of soap, detergent, or other materials used in the genital area.

7. Modifying Your Lifestyle Eating a nutritious, well-balanced diet and getting regular exercise will help you stay in good health and lower your risk of developing balanitis and other related illnesses.

8. Conservative management of balanitis requires regular check-ins with a healthcare physician to assess whether or not the condition is improving. The treatment plan can be modified as needed.

If you suspect you have balanitis, see a doctor to get a proper diagnosis and advice on the most effective non-invasive treatments for your condition. More complex therapies may be necessary, and your doctor will discuss these options with you if conservative management fails to alleviate your symptoms or if issues arise.

Alternative Treatments

Balanitis can be brought on by anything from an infection to an irritant, therefore treating it is condition-specific. The following are examples of typical balanitis treatments:

1. In mild cases, better cleanliness is frequently the first line of defense. To avoid smegma buildup, it is recommended to regularly wash the genital area with warm water and mild soap.

2. Creams and Lotions:

- Balanitis caused by a fungal infection (candidal balanitis) is typically treated with antifungal creams like clotrimazole or miconazole. Follow the indicated course of treatment.

Oral antibiotics and antibiotic lotions for the skin may be recommended for bacterial infections.

3. Skin-Applying Steroids:

• Balanitis is characterized by irritation and itching, and in some situations, topical corticosteroid creams may be prescribed to alleviate these symptoms.

4. Drugs taken via mouth:

• Oral antifungal or antibiotic drugs may be administered for more severe or resistant instances. These are frequently used in tandem with topical therapies.

5. Resolving Root Causes:

• To properly manage balanitis, it is necessary to treat the underlying medical condition that is causing it, such as diabetes or a skin issue.

6. When various therapies for balanitis, including antibiotics, steroids, and rest, fail, a doctor may consider circumcision to remove the foreskin and lessen the likelihood of future flare-ups.

7. Dealing with Triggers and Allergens:

• Determining and avoiding irritants and allergens is essential if contact dermatitis is to blame. Changing the type of soap, detergent, or other products used in the genital area may be necessary.

8. How to Treat Phimosis

• Gentle stretching exercises and the application of topical steroid creams may help soften the foreskin if phimosis (a tight foreskin) is a factor in balanitis. Circumcision is sometimes advised.

9. After-Care Services:

• If you're currently receiving medical treatment, it's crucial that you schedule follow-up appointments so that your doctor can check in on your recovery. They'll be able to monitor your progress and make adjustments to your treatment accordingly.

10. Recurrence Avoidance:

• Balanitis can be prevented by practicing proper genital cleanliness, switching to looser-fitting underwear, and avoiding known irritants and allergens that bring on flare-ups.

A healthcare provider should evaluate and diagnose balanitis to decide the best course of treatment. Untreated or persistent balanitis can cause difficulties and discomfort, so it's important to get medical care if you experience any symptoms. In addition, there may be variations in treatment based on the etiology and the specifics of each patient's case.

CHAPTER FOUR
Balanitis Precautions

Balanitis can be avoided by practicing safe sexual behavior and taking other measures to prevent genital infections and irritations. Some suggestions for warding off balanitis:

1. Keeping a Routine:

• Clean the genital area, including the glans and under the foreskin (if present), regularly with warm water and mild, unscented soap. Dry everything completely afterward.

2. Put away Dangerous Goods

• Use mild, non-irritating soaps and detergents for washing your genital area. Scented and perfumed goods should be avoided because of their unpleasant effects.

3. Maintaining Healthy Foreskin:

• If you are not circumcised, your foreskin should be retracted gently while washing and returned to its normal place thereafter. The foreskin is easily torn and inflamed if you pull on it too roughly.

4. Get Away From Stimulants:

• Avoid using strong soaps, laundry detergents, or topical creams with scents or allergies, since these can all irritate the skin and aggravate balanitis symptoms. Pick hypoallergenic options instead.

5. Put on Loose Clothes:

• Choose underwear and clothing that is loose fitting to increase airflow and decrease genital area friction.

6. To prevent STIs, which can lead to balanitis, it is recommended to always use a condom when engaging in sexual activity.

7. Stay away from sexually risky behaviors:

• Reduce your risk of sexually transmitted infections by limiting the number of people with whom you have s*x and only using safe sexual practices.

8. Take Care of the Root Cause:

• Working closely with your doctor is essential if you suffer from a condition that raises your risk of balanitis, such as diabetes or a skin disorder.

9. Balanitis is a complication of urinary tract infections, which can be avoided with regular water intake.

10. Routine Medical Exams:

• Keep up with your regular checkups so that you can keep tabs on your health and identify any potential problems in their early stages.

11. Circumcision:

• Recurrent or severe balanitis may warrant serious consideration of circumcision. Consult your doctor about the pros and cons of circumcision.

Balanitis can be avoided with preventative measures, but if you notice any redness, swelling, itching, or discharge in the genital area, you should consult a doctor right away. When balanitis is diagnosed and treated promptly, problems can be avoided and pain can be reduced.

Sustaining Balanitis

Balanitis can be difficult to manage, especially if the symptoms are causing you pain and frustration. Here are some methods that have helped others deal with balanitis:

• Seek Professional Help If you experience balanitis symptoms or think you might have balanitis, you should see a doctor to get a proper diagnosis and treatment plan. They can explain the problem and provide you advice on how to handle it.

• Do as your doctor tells you and finish the course of treatment they've set out for you. Treatments might range from simple lifestyle adjustments to surgical procedures. Consistency in treatment is necessary for the best outcomes.

• To avoid further irritation and infection, keep up with your regular hygienic routine. Warm water and gentle soap applied on a regular basis will ease soreness and speed recovery.

• **Avoid Irritants:** Be diligent about avoiding irritants that may cause balanitis. Products with strong fragrances or allergies fall into this category. Choose items that are hypoallergenic and odorless.

• Choose loose-fitting underwear and apparel to reduce the risk of chafing and to maximize airflow. This can help minimize inflammation in the vaginal area.

• If your balanitis was caused by a sexually transmitted illness, you can lessen the likelihood of reinfection by using condoms and sticking to monogamous relationships.

• The stress of dealing with balanitis and its symptoms should be minimized. To better handle stress and pain, try engaging in stress-reduction activities like meditation, deep breathing, or physical activity.

• If your health is interfering with your sexual life or your intimate relationships, talking to your partner about it can help you both cope.

• **Follow Up Appointments:** It's important to keep up with your doctor's follow-up appointments so that he or she may check in on your progress and make any required adjustments to your therapy.

• Consider joining a local support group, either online or in person, where you may connect with others who are dealing with the same issues.

• Learn more about balanitis and what might be triggering it. Once you have a firm grasp of the condition, you will be better equipped to deal with it and avoid further instances.

• **Patience:** Balanitis can take time to resolve, depending on its cause and severity. Maintain your treatment and good habits while waiting.

Keep in mind that balanitis is a medically manageable ailment from which the vast majority of people can recover with the correct treatment and attention. Please see your doctor if you have any questions or concerns about your illness or treatment plan, especially if your symptoms worsen or persist.

Conclusion

Infections, poor hygiene, irritants, and underlying medical disorders are just some of the many potential triggers for balanitis, or inflammation of the glans penis. Redness, swelling, itching, and pain in the vaginal area are common manifestations. Conservative treatments and medical procedures, such as topical medicines and, in extremely rare situations, circumcision, are effective against balanitis.

- Balanitis can be avoided by practicing proper genital hygiene, staying away from potential irritants, and decreasing the likelihood of infection. In order to have an accurate diagnosis and effective treatment, it is crucial to visit a doctor as soon as possible after experiencing symptoms.

• Balanitis can be difficult to live with, but it is manageable with the help of a healthcare provider, consistent medication use, and careful attention to personal hygiene.

Always seek the advice of a medical expert for the most accurate diagnosis and the most effective course of treatment and prevention of balanitis, as each individual case is different. The majority of people who suffer from balanitis can get well once they receive treatment.

THE END